J
BIOG
MURRAY

Mattern, Joanne,
1963-

Joseph E. Murray and
the story of the
first human kidney
transplant.

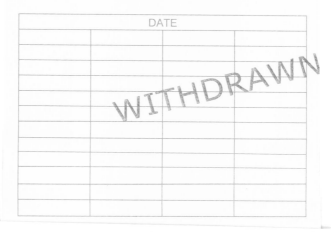

DATE			

WITHDRAWN

Joseph E. Murray and the Story of the First Human Kidney Transplant

Joanne Mattern

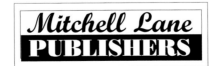

Mitchell Lane
PUBLISHERS

PO Box 619 • Bear, Delaware 19701
www.mitchelllane.com

Unlocking the Secrets of Science

Profiling 20th Century Achievers in Science, Medicine, and Technology

Joseph E. Murray and the Story of the First Human Kidney Transplant

• •

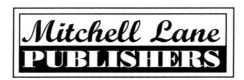

Copyright © 2003 by Mitchell Lane Publishers, Inc. All rights reserved. No part of this book may be reproduced without written permission from the publisher. Printed and bound in the United States of America.

Printing   1   2   3   4   5   6   7   8   9   10

Library of Congress Cataloging-in-Publication Data

Mattern, Joanne, 1963-
     Joseph E. Murray and the story of the first human kidney transplant/Joanne Mattern.
        p. cm. — (Unlocking the secrets of science)
     Summary: A biography of the American surgeon who received the Nobel Prize in Medicine for his work on kidney transplants.
     Includes bibliographical references and index.
     ISBN 1-58415-136-6 (lib. bdg.)
     1. Murray, Joseph E., 1919—Juvenile literature. 2. Transplant surgeons—United States—Biography—Juvenile literature. 3. Kidneys—Transplantation—Juvenile literature. 4. Kidneys—Transplantation. [1. Murray, Joseph E., 1919- 2. Physicians. 3. Nobel Prizes—Biography.] I. Title. II. Series.
RD27.35.M875 M38 2003
617.9'5'092—dc21
    [B]   2002066127

ABOUT THE AUTHOR: Joanne Mattern is the author of more than 100 nonfiction books for children. Along with biographies, she has written extensively about animals, nature, history, sports, and foreign cultures. She lives near New York City with her husband and two young daughters.

CHILDREN'S SCIENCE REVIEW EDITOR: Stephanie Kondrchek, B.S. Microbiology, University of Maryland

PHOTO CREDITS: cover: National Archives of Plastic Surgery/Francis A. Countway Library of Medicine; p. 6 Hulton/Getty; pp. 10, 14, 21, 22, 26, 34, 40 National Archives of Plastic Surgery/Francis A. Countway Library of Medicine; p. 19 Corbis; p. 28 AP Photo

PUBLISHER'S NOTE: In selecting those persons to be profiled in this series, we first attempted to identify the most notable accomplishments of the 20th century in science, medicine, and technology. When we were done, we noted a serious deficiency in the inclusion of women. For the greater part of the 20th century science, medicine, and technology were male-dominated fields. In many cases, the contributions of women went unrecognized. Women have tried for years to be included in these areas, and in many cases, women worked side by side with men who took credit for their ideas and discoveries. Even as we move forward into the 21st century, we find women still sadly underrepresented. It is not an oversight, therefore, that we profiled mostly male achievers. Information simply does not exist to include a fair selection of women.

Contents

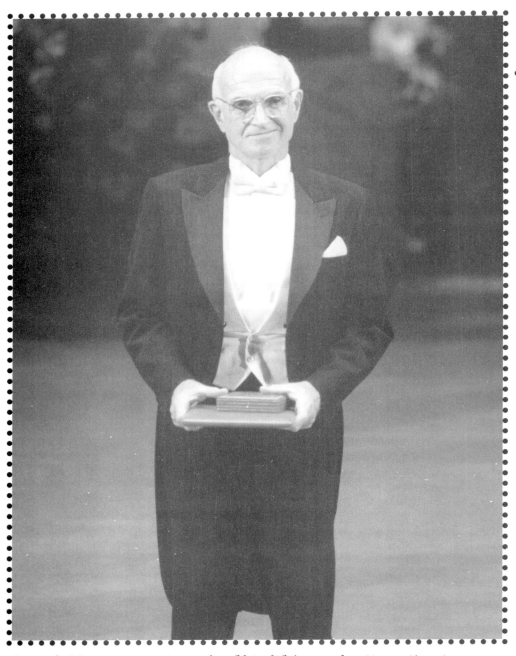

Joseph Murray spent much of his life's work attempting to overcome the body's natural reaction to reject foreign tissues. His work eventually led to the first successful kidney transplant, for which he won a Nobel Prize in 1990.

Chapter 1

Creating a New Face

• •

The year 1945 was a frightening and exciting time to be a surgeon. The United States was fighting in World War II. American soldiers were stationed all over Europe, in the Pacific Ocean, and in Asia. Many of these soldiers suffered terrible injuries in battle. When their injuries were too serious to be treated at hospitals near the battlefields, they were sent back to the United States for medical help. Doctors at American hospitals faced injuries more serious than they had ever seen before.

Many American soldiers found their way to Valley Forge General Hospital in Phoenixville, Pennsylvania. One of the doctors there was a 25-year-old surgeon named Joseph Murray. He was just beginning his medical career, and he was about to meet a patient who would change his life. This patient was a young pilot named Charles Woods.

Woods was only 22 years old. During takeoff in Burma (a country southwest of China that is now known as Myanmar), his plane crashed and exploded. Woods escaped, but 70 percent of his body had been terribly burned. His face and hands were destroyed.

Doctors in Burma could not provide care for Woods, so they sent him back to the United States. Woods was so sick, he could travel for only a few days at a time. It took six weeks for him to reach Valley Forge.

When Murray first saw Woods, he couldn't believe the pilot had survived the long, difficult journey to the hospital. Woods was barely alive.

Burns are one of the most serious injuries a person can suffer. Burned skin cannot hold fluids, so the body quickly becomes dehydrated. Burns are also extremely painful and easily become infected.

Murray and the other doctors knew that they had to cover Woods' burned skin with new, healthy skin. New skin would prevent infection and fluid loss. The doctors found this new skin by taking skin from the unburned parts of Woods' body. They placed the undamaged skin on the burned areas. These skin grafts—grafts from the same body—are called autografts.

Woods had so many burns that he did not have enough healthy skin to cover them all. Also, removing healthy skin meant undergoing surgery, and Woods was too sick to have these operations. The doctors decided to use skin from a dead body, a cadaver. This type of skin graft—a graft taken from another person—is called an allograft.

Allografts do not work as well as autografts because the body naturally rejects foreign tissue. After about two weeks, the grafted skin shrinks and falls off. However, using allografts on Woods gave the pilot time to get stronger. Later, doctors were able to use autografts.

Over the next few months, Woods had many operations to replace his burned skin. Murray used tweezers to place tiny squares of new skin on Woods' hands and face. Later, Woods had more surgery to reconstruct his destroyed face and hands. Twenty-four operations and one and a half years later, Woods was finally able to go home.

Charles Woods became one of the most important patients in Joseph Murray's career. Before treating Woods,

Murray had never worked with skin grafts. He was fascinated by the fact that the body rejected skin from another person. Why did this happen? How could it be prevented? If rejection could be stopped, could other parts of the body besides skin be transplanted?

Murray spent much of his career addressing these questions. His work led to the first successful human kidney transplant. And it helped change the lives of thousands of people all over the world.

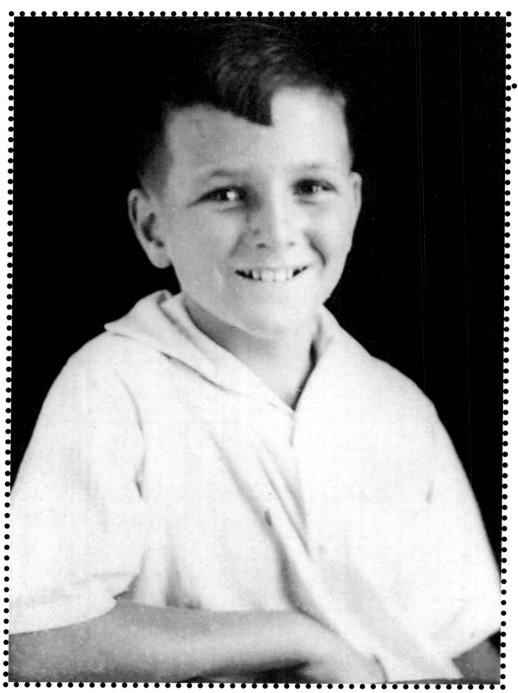

Even as a child, Joseph Murray knew he wanted to be a surgeon.

Chapter 2

Life in Milford

• •

Joseph E. Murray was born on April 1, 1919, in Milford, Massachusetts. Milford was a small town about 30 miles southwest of Boston. Joseph's father, William, was Irish, and his mother, Mary DePasquale Murray, was Italian. Joseph was the baby of the family. He had an older sister, Mary Norma, and an older brother, William, Jr.

William Murray, Sr., was a lawyer who loved to read. Sunday night was his reading night. His favorite subjects were history, biography, and classic literature from ancient Greece and Rome. As he got older, Joseph often shared his father's reading night. "We had wonderful discussions on as many topics as we had books in our library," he later recalled in his autobiography, *Surgery of the Soul.*

Mary Murray had worked as a teacher and a clerk in her husband's law office. She was also very active in politics and was honored by the Massachusetts Legislature for her contributions to the state.

Both William and Mary wanted their children to be good citizens. Joseph recalls many times when his father worked for free to help poor people solve legal problems or fill out complicated government forms. Mary took her children to visit patients in hospitals and mental institutions. His parents' example taught Joseph to care for other people and always do his best to help them.

Education was also important in the Murray family. Joseph attended Milford's public schools from elementary through high school. He knew that he needed an education for the career he had chosen. Even when he was a small child, he knew exactly what he wanted to do with his life: he wanted to be a surgeon.

After he graduated from high school, Murray attended the College of the Holy Cross. In 1940 he graduated with honors and was accepted into Harvard Medical School.

Being a medical student was a tremendous amount of work. But life at Harvard was also a lot of fun. Murray and his friends enjoyed sports and music. Murray often went to parties and to concerts by the Boston Symphony Orchestra.

At one of these concerts, Murray met a young woman named Virginia Link, whom everyone called Bobby. Bobby was actually dating one of Murray's friends, but Murray didn't let that stop him. "That night back in my room in Vanderbilt Hall I announced to my roommate that I had met the girl I would marry," Murray wrote in *Surgery of the Soul.* He was right. On June 2, 1945, Joseph and Bobby married in a small ceremony near her family's home in upstate New York.

Before he married Bobby, however, Murray had to finish school. When the United States entered World War II on December 7, 1941, Murray's life became even more complicated. Every medical student was automatically drafted into the armed forces. Murray wanted to join the Navy, but he was too nearsighted to qualify. Instead he joined the Army. Murray remained at Harvard Medical School, but his training was accelerated so that he could enter military service as soon as possible.

From 1941 to 1943, Murray went to classes. He also worked as a surgical intern at Peter Bent Brigham Hospital (now Brigham and Women's Hospital) in Boston. There, he treated patients and worked with other doctors on many different medical cases.

In December 1943, Murray completed medical school. It was time to see where the U.S. Army would send him. Murray reported to Fort Dix, New Jersey, and waited in line to hear where he would start his medical career. Everyone ahead of him was assigned to duty overseas. Murray was engaged to Bobby at the time, and he really wanted to stay in the United States so that he could be near her.

Then something surprising happened. Just as he stepped up to the desk, the officer on duty received a phone call. After a brief conversation, the officer told Murray that an assignment had just come in from Valley Forge General Hospital in Pennsylvania. Was he interested?

Murray could not believe his good luck. He told the officer that he was *very* interested in the job. His assignment to Valley Forge would change Murray's life—and the world of medicine—forever.

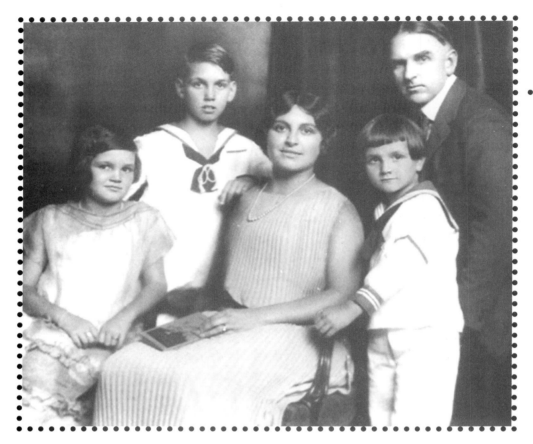

William and Mary Murray, with their three children, including Joseph (right), Mary Norma (left), and William, Jr. (back). The Murray family were avid readers and both William and Mary wanted their children to be good citizens. His parents raised Joseph to care for other people and always do his best to help them.

14

Chapter 3
Learning on the Job

• •

V alley Forge General Hospital was one of eight hospitals in the United States that specialized in plastic and reconstructive surgery. Like Charles Woods, many of the patients at Valley Forge were soldiers who had been badly burned or injured in battle. Joseph Murray learned on the job, both from his patients and from the other doctors on the unit.

From one moment to the next, he never knew what to expect. In *Surgery of the Soul,* Murray recalls, "Severe cases were the norm. Hundreds of patients arrived with every . . . type of injury. The daily operating schedules were chock full of exciting challenges: bone grafts to jaws and skulls; restoration of eyelids, ears, and noses; repair of ulcers."

Despite the challenges of working at Valley Forge, Murray wanted to go back to Boston. He especially wanted to work at Peter Bent Brigham Hospital, where he had done some of his training. However, the Army kept Murray at Valley Forge even after the war ended in August 1945. Many injured soldiers were still being sent there, and Murray and other doctors were needed to take care of them.

Finally, in 1947, Murray was released from military service. He returned to Brigham as an assistant resident in surgery. He also worked for six months at Memorial Hospital in New York City as part of an exchange program. Memorial Hospital was a major cancer center. While he worked there, Murray performed many operations to remove cancerous tumors from patients' heads, faces, and necks. He also reconstructed their damaged bodies through plastic surgery.

In 1951 Murray completed his medical training. He had decided to be a plastic surgeon because he received so much joy and satisfaction from helping patients improve their lives. However, he had other interests as well.

Ever since he helped care for Charles Woods at Valley Forge, Murray had been interested in why the body rejects transplanted skin and other organs. When he began working at Boston's Brigham Hospital, he found out that George Thorn, the physician in chief at Brigham, had started a kidney transplant program. This program allowed Murray to research the problem of transplant rejection.

The kidneys are two reddish brown, kidney bean–shaped organs that are located on either side of the spine, just below the diaphragm. These organs have three important jobs: they regulate the amount of water in the body, produce vital hormones, and remove liquid waste from the body. Almost everyone is born with two kidneys.

Filtering waste and other toxins out of the body is one of the kidneys' most important jobs. One of the waste products is urea, which is a result of the breakdown of proteins, such as meat, by the digestive system. Another waste product is creatinine, which comes from the activity of the muscles.

The kidneys also balance the amount of minerals in the body. Some minerals, such as sodium and potassium, are necessary to stay healthy, but having too much of them in the bloodstream can be toxic.

After the kidneys remove toxins from the bloodstream, they change these wastes into a liquid called urine. Urine travels through a tube called the ureter into the bladder, where it is excreted from the body. A person who has damaged kidneys cannot remove waste from his or her body. These wastes build up and poison the body. In time, the person will die from the buildup of toxins.

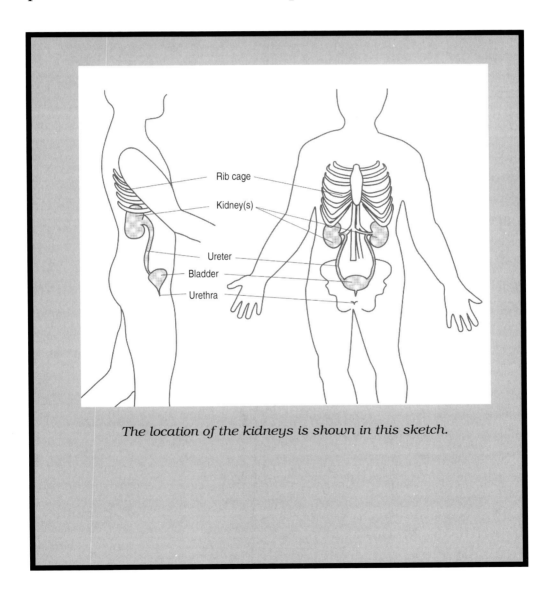

The location of the kidneys is shown in this sketch.

Many things can damage a person's kidneys. Sometimes the organs become infected. Some infections are acute, which means they occur suddenly. Others are chronic, which means a person may have them for many years. Kidneys can also be damaged by diabetes, high blood pressure, poisoning such as by alcohol or a drug overdose, or an injury. Some kidney diseases and defects are hereditary, passed from parent to child.

During the 1940s, a Dutch doctor named Willem Kolff designed an artificial kidney called a dialysis machine. A dialysis machine takes blood out of the body and removes wastes from it, then sends the blood back into the body. Although this procedure could prolong people's lives, it was not easy. A person on dialysis had to spend many hours hooked up to the machine. Because the body constantly produces waste, the dialysis treatment had to be repeated every few days.

George Thorn knew there had to be a better way to help patients with kidney disease. What if doctors could transplant a healthy kidney into a patient to do the work the damaged kidneys couldn't? These donor kidneys could be taken from cadavers. They could even be taken from living donors. The body only needs one kidney, so a person with two healthy kidneys could donate one and still live a normal life.

However, there were many problems with the idea of transplanting an organ. The biggest problem was rejection. The human body is always on the lookout for invaders that might be harmful. If a foreign organism is found, the body's immune system fights to remove the invader. If a transplanted organ is rejected, it will stop working and be destroyed by the body's immune system. Patients can also suffer a condition called graft-versus-host disease, which is an overreaction by the immune system that can kill the patient. For these reasons, if foreign tissue—in this case, the transplanted organ—is rejected, it must be removed.

There were other problems to consider as well. Transplanting an organ meant cutting off its blood supply. Without fresh blood, the organ could survive for only a short time. Doctors had to attach the organ to the new blood supply as quickly as possible. Nerve endings also had to be attached. These were all complicated surgical procedures that no one had ever tried to do.

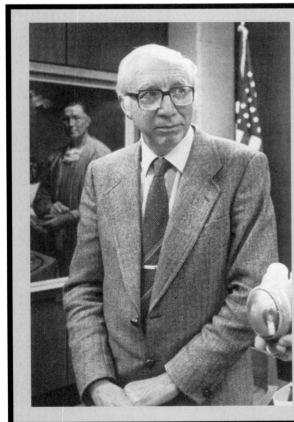

Willem Kolff designed an artificial kidney called a dialysis machine. The machine can prolong a person's life, but it is not easy. A person on dialysis must spend many hours hooked up to a machine.

When Murray heard about the kidney transplant program at Brigham, he couldn't wait to join. He knew that the body would reject a kidney for the same reason that it rejected a skin graft. However, not everyone shared Murray's enthusiasm. "At that time, the concept of organ transplantation was so revolutionary that it was generally deemed not worth pursuing," he recalled in his autobiography. "One of my closest friends, a professor at Harvard Medical School, took me aside and said, 'Joe, don't get involved in that. It will never work, and you may ruin your whole future.'"

Murray didn't listen to his friend. Instead, he joined the program and began doing research and conducting experiments. Soon he was put in charge of the experiments that were being done to figure out how to successfully transplant kidneys.

Many of Murray's early experiments were done on dogs. At that time, no dogs had survived very long with a transplanted kidney. Murray operated on many dogs to discover the best place to put a transplanted kidney. He also learned how to connect important tissues, nerves, and blood vessels so that the kidney would work in its new body.

Murray's work would not have been possible without the discoveries of a French physician named Alexis Carrel. Carrel paved the way for organ transplants when he discovered a way to rejoin severed blood vessels. This allowed surgeons to remove an organ and reconnect the arteries and veins to a new, transplanted organ. In 1912, Carrel won the Nobel Prize in medicine for his work.

Another breakthrough was the discovery of heparin in 1937. Heparin is an anticoagulant, or a substance that prevents blood from clotting. When heparin is injected into a patient, the person's blood will not clot when it stops flowing. This was a tremendous help to surgeons who needed to stop blood flow temporarily during an operation.

By the summer of 1954, several dogs in Murray's laboratory had survived for years with transplanted kidneys. All of these transplants were autografts. The doctors had removed a dog's kidney, then put it back into the same dog's body. Murray and the other doctors still had not been able to solve the problem of a body rejecting a kidney from a donor. However, they were ready to try a kidney transplant on humans. How could they perform such a transplant without the risk that the organ would be rejected?

The answer came a few months later. That's when Murray met a pair of identical twins named Richard and Ronald Herrick.

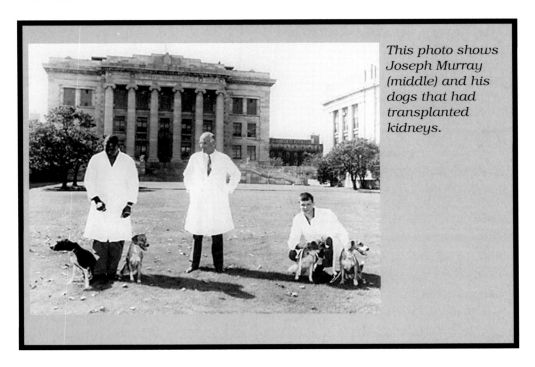

This photo shows Joseph Murray (middle) and his dogs that had transplanted kidneys.

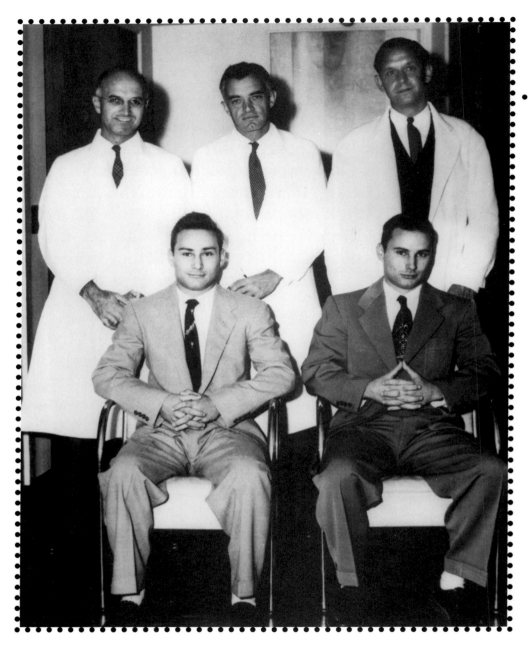

The Herrick twins and their doctors (Joseph Murray on left). In October of 1954, Richard Herrick was dying of chronic nephritis. His brother Ronald agreed to donate a healthy kidney to Richard, who lived for eight years after the surgery.

Chapter 4
Identical Kidneys

· ·

Identical twins look exactly alike. Their bodies are also exactly alike. The tissues, organs, blood, and everything else inside their bodies are the same. Joseph Murray and the other doctors at Brigham thought that if a person donated a kidney to his identical twin, the organ would not be rejected because it was exactly like the kidney in the patient's own body.

Murray got the chance to test this idea late in 1954. On October 26, Richard Herrick was admitted to Brigham Hospital. He was only 23 years old, but he was dying of chronic nephritis, a life-threatening inflammation of the kidneys. The only things keeping him alive were dialysis, a number of medications, and the careful control of the fluid balance in his body. Despite these steps, Richard's kidneys were so damaged that he did not have long to live. His identical twin brother, Ronald, agreed to donate one of his healthy kidneys to save Richard's life.

Before the brothers could be accepted into the transplant program, doctors had to make sure they really were identical. The twins had 17 different genetic tests, including fingerprinting and skin grafts. All the tests proved that the two men really were identical.

There were other problems to solve before the doctors could go ahead with the transplant. The biggest worry was whether taking a healthy kidney out of a person's body was ethical. In his Nobel Prize lecture many years later, Murray talked about this issue. "For the first time in medical history a normal healthy person was to be subjected to a major surgical operation not for his own benefit."

Murray talked to other doctors, lawyers, and members of the clergy before he felt he could do the operation. In addition, he made sure the Herrick brothers and their family also talked to doctors and counselors so that they would understand what they were about to do.

Although he wanted to help his brother, Ronald Herrick had serious doubts about the transplant. "I had heard of such things, but it seemed in the realm of science fiction," Murray's autobiography quoted Ronald Herrick as saying. "When it became clear that Richard would die without one of my kidneys, I did some serious soul-searching. I mean, here I was, 23 years old, young and healthy, and they were going to cut me open and take out one of my organs. It was shocking even to consider the idea. I felt a real conflict of emotions. Of course I wanted to help my brother, but the only operation I'd ever had before was an appendectomy, and I hadn't much liked that."

Finally, Ronald agreed. The operation was scheduled for December 23. By then, the story of what Murray was going to try to do was big news all over the world. As he drove to the hospital that morning, he heard reporters talking about the operation on the radio.

The surgery began at 8:15 in the morning. By 9:50, Ronald Herrick's healthy kidney was ready to be removed. Three minutes later, the kidney was wrapped in a cold, wet towel and sitting in a basin. When surgeons took out the donor organ, they also cut off its blood supply. Without fresh blood, the kidney would soon die. Murray and the other doctors had to get Richard Herrick's body ready to receive the kidney as quickly as possible.

While one team of surgeons worked on Ronald to reconnect the blood vessels inside his body and close the surgical incision, Murray and another team prepared Richard for the transplant. They cut the blood vessels and nerves that ran in and out of his damaged kidneys. Then they carefully placed Ronald's donor kidney into Richard's body and reattached all the nerves, veins, arteries, and other vessels. One hour and 22 minutes later, blood began to flow into the donated kidney. The organ quickly turned pink and urine began to flow out of it. The kidney was working.

Murray finished the operation by attaching Richard's ureter and bladder to the new kidney so that urine could leave the body normally. Finally, the operation was finished.

Even though the operation had gone very well, doctors would not know for several weeks if it had been a success. During that time, they watched Richard carefully to make sure that his kidney continued to work properly. They also checked for signs that would indicate whether Richard's body had become infected or was rejecting the organ. They also monitored Ronald to make sure his remaining kidney was working properly, and that he didn't suffer any infections or other ill effects from the surgery. Fortunately, no problems occurred to either twin. Five weeks after the operation, both Ronald and Richard were well enough to go home.

Richard's old, damaged kidneys had been left in his body. Murray wanted to remove them during the transplant surgery to cut down on the chances that the kidney disease

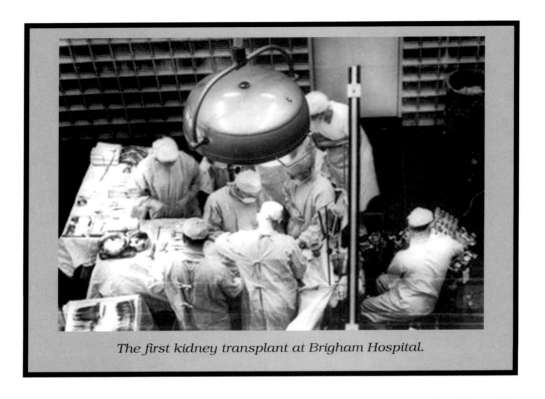

The first kidney transplant at Brigham Hospital.

would spread to the new organs. However, John P. Merrill, who was the head of the kidney transplant unit, disagreed. He thought that the old organs should remain in the body in case the new kidney failed. Damaged organs were better than no organs at all, and having his old kidneys in his body might give Richard some extra time should something happen to the new kidney.

Richard's diseased left kidney was finally removed on March 29, 1955. His right kidney was removed on June 20, 1955. Richard Herrick lived for eight years with his new kidney. He died in 1962 because the chronic nephritis that had damaged his original kidneys destroyed the donor kidney.

After performing several more transplants and studying the results, Merrill agreed with Murray that it was better to remove the diseased kidneys during the transplant. When this was done, the donor kidney usually remained healthy.

After the successful surgery, Murray, the other doctors of the transplant team, and the Herrick twins became famous around the world. The operation showed doctors, scientists, and kidney patients that transplants really could save lives.

However, there was one problem with the Herrick operation. Because it had been performed on identical twins, doctors didn't have to worry about the recipient's body rejecting the organ. But rejection was still a serious threat in kidney transplants between patients who were not identical twins. The Herrick operation had been a huge step forward, but there was still a great deal of work to be done.

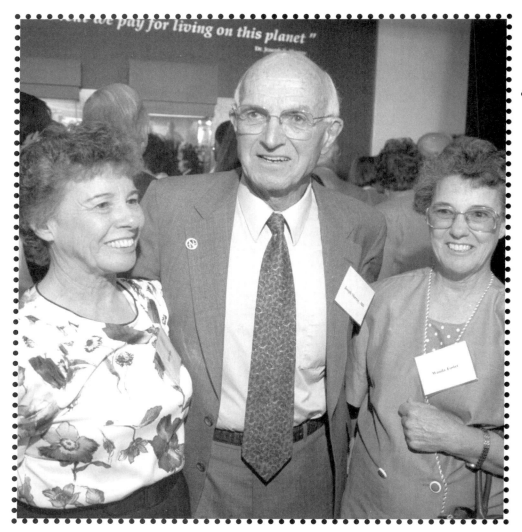

Though Murray didn't think that he would perform many transplants on identical twins, he was surprised to find that he performed one or two every year. In May 1956, Murray performed a kidney transplant for Edith Helm (shown here on left) using the kidney of her twin sister, Wanda Foster (right). Helm went on to be the longest living transplant recipient. The two women lived for more than 45 years after their operations.

Chapter 5

Tricking the Body

● ●

Joseph Murray didn't think that he would perform many more kidney transplants on identical twins. He felt the Herrick brothers had been an unusual case. To his surprise, he performed one or two of these operations every year.

In May 1956, Murray performed a kidney transplant for Edith Helm using a kidney from her identical twin, Wanda Foster. Helm went on to become the longest-lived transplant recipient, and the first recipient to become pregnant and have children. Foster also had successful pregnancies, despite having only one kidney. The two women lived for more than 45 years after their operations.

While identical-twin transplant surgery was a success, Murray knew that most people could not benefit from this operation. Along with other doctors and scientists, Murray began experimenting with ways to suppress or destroy the body's immune system so that it wouldn't reject the transplanted organ.

The human immune system protects the body from invading organisms called antigens. An antigen can be a virus, bacteria, a foreign object (such as a splinter), or a collection of strange cells (such as an organ transplant). One of the major parts of the immune system is white blood cells. These special cells attack antigens and destroy them.

If a person's immune system were suppressed, it would not react as strongly to invaders. In a transplant patient, this would allow a transplanted organ to function without being attacked and destroyed. Unfortunately, a suppressed immune system also would not resist other foreign objects, such as germs. This meant that the transplant patient would be likely to die from infection. For example, if the patient cut his finger, bacteria could enter the body and cause a life-threatening condition.

As he had done before, Murray began his experiments on dogs. At first he had no success. Then he heard about a doctor named John Mannick who was working in a hospital in Cooperstown, New York. Mannick also worked with dogs. He would give a dog huge doses of radiation to destroy all its white blood cells. This procedure was called total-body irradiation. Then Mannick would replace the dog's bone marrow so that it could produce new blood and a new immune system. He hoped that the new immune system would not reject the transplanted kidney.

Murray and the other doctors at Brigham tried Mannick's procedure on dogs. Although the patients did well at first, their bodies always rejected the transplanted kidneys after a few weeks.

During this time, Murray also tried the radiation procedure on human patients. His first patient was Gladys Loman, a 31-year-old woman who was born with only one kidney. The kidney became infected and was mistakenly removed by a doctor, who thought it was her appendix. Without any kidneys, Loman was doomed. She agreed to try Murray's experimental procedure.

Loman was treated with total-body irradiation to destroy her immune system. Then she had a kidney transplant. At first her transplant didn't function properly. Finally, after two weeks, the kidney began producing urine. Unfortunately, a month later, Loman caught an infection. Without a working immune system, her body was unable to fight back, and she died.

Murray and his team of doctors performed several more transplants using total-body irradiation. Only one of their patients survived. His name was John Riteris. Riteris was 24 years old and suffering from kidney disease. He received a kidney from his fraternal twin brother, Andrew. Although identical twins are completely alike in every physical way, fraternal twins are not. Because John and Andrew were not identical twins, the transplant had little chance of success.

About 10 days after the transplant, John came down with a serious infection. He almost died. Somehow his body fought off the infection and he survived. Riteris lived for 29 more years with his transplanted kidney.

Murray was thrilled at the success of John Riteris' operation. Another transplant surgeon, Thomas Starzl, later wrote in the *Journal of NIH Research* that this transplant was "the single most important case, psychologically and otherwise, in the history of the field of clinical transplantation."

Unfortunately, Murray and other surgeons did not have the same success with other patients. It was clear they had to try something new.

In 1959 Murray read an article in a magazine called *Nature.* This article described how two doctors at Tufts

Medical School in Boston had done experiments with an anticancer drug called 6-mercaptopurine, or 6-MP. Using 6-MP, the doctors had tricked the immune systems of rabbits. When they injected a foreign protein into the rabbits' bodies along with the 6-MP, the rabbits' bodies did not react against the protein. However, the rabbits' immune systems still worked and fought against other foreign organisms in their bodies.

Murray was very excited to hear about these experiments. Working with other doctors, he administered 6-MP and another drug, Imuran, to the dogs in his laboratory. Imuran is a drug that prevents rejection by disrupting the growth of white blood cells.

Murray's experiments were a success. When dogs received the drugs along with a kidney transplant, they survived for months, and then years. After one dog survived for 1,000 days (almost three years), the doctors and lab workers tied a ribbon around the dog's neck and threw a party. The best news was that the dogs didn't just survive the operation. They were healthy and happy and could live normal lives.

In 1961 Murray began using Imuran with kidney transplants on humans. At first he did not have the same success with people as he'd had with dogs. The biggest problem was figuring out how much Imuran to give the patient. Several times the dose was too high, and the patients' immune systems were too badly damaged to recover. In other cases, the kidney transplant failed.

Then, on April 5, 1962, Murray operated on a man named Mel Doucette. Doucette was a 23-year-old accountant. His kidney transplant happened because of a coincidence. While Doucette was at Brigham for a dialysis treatment, another man who was having open-heart surgery died on the operating table. Tests showed that the dead man's blood type was the same as Doucette's. After getting permission from the dead man's family and talking things over with Doucette, the doctors went ahead and performed the kidney transplant that night.

Once again, Murray and the other doctors struggled to decide how much Imuran to give Doucette. Murray argued for a small dose of only two to four milligrams. Merrill, the head of the kidney transplant program, wanted to give Doucette a higher dosage. He also recommended small doses of radiation to weaken Doucette's immune system. Murray later wrote in *Surgery of the Soul*, "We had honest differences of opinion about the type and amount of drug to use and whether the drug should be supplemented by radiation…We knew all too well that the wrong decision could cost the patient his life."

Finally, Merrill agreed to Murray's plan. The transplant was a complete success and Doucette survived for many years. Recalling the earlier celebration for the dog that survived 1,000 days, Murray commented in his autobiography that when Doucette "reached the one-year mark, we refrained from tying a ribbon around his neck." Instead, in June 1963, Murray, Merrill, and the other doctors who had worked with Doucette reported their success in the *New England Journal of Medicine*. From then on, organ transplants would never be the same.

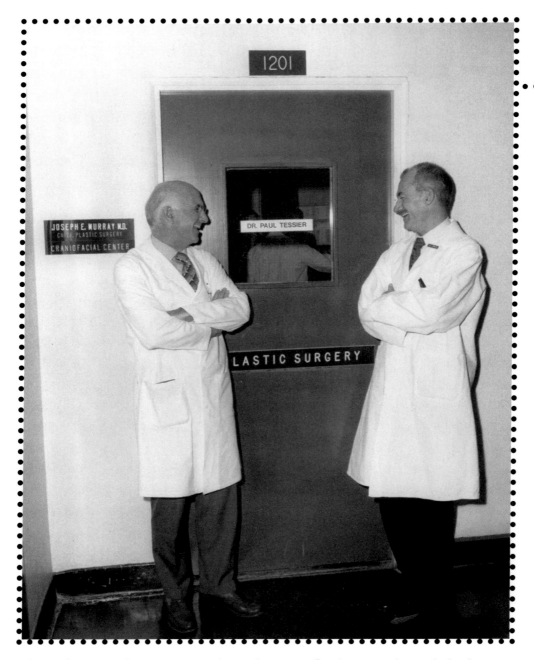

Though Joseph Murray is best known for his work with kidney transplants, he worked as a plastic surgeon all his life. Many of his patients were children who suffered from severe deformities. He is shown here with Paul Tessier.

Chapter 6
Changing Paths

• •

After Mel Doucette's successful transplant in 1962, Joseph Murray remained an important figure in kidney transplants. In 1963 he was one of the organizers of an international conference on human kidney transplants. This conference was held in Washington, D.C. Doctors and scientists came from all over the United States, as well as from England, Scotland, France, Germany, and Denmark.

The scientists at the conference shared their information and experiences with transplants. They also decided to come up with specific standards for kidney transplants. Because every doctor had his own way of doing things, it was hard to compare results and make sure that every patient was receiving the best possible care. The National Kidney Registry was formed to solve this problem. Soon almost every hospital in the world was following the same procedures and reporting their results directly to Murray and his team at Brigham. During the 1970s, the program became so large that Murray could not administer it any longer. Instead, the American College of Surgeons took over the job for a few years. Then the U.S. government stepped in to run the program.

Although Murray was thrilled and excited about his work in kidney transplants, he continued to work as a plastic surgeon. While he was researching and performing transplants, he was also removing tumors from patients' faces and necks. Many of his patients suffered from cancer.

Others were disabled or disfigured by birth defects or accidents.

Many of Murray's patients were children. He found it especially rewarding to save a child from death, and then to make it possible for the child to live a normal life.

Murray practiced medicine not just in Boston. He also made trips to other countries. In 1962 he spent two months working at the Christian Medical School in Vellore, India. He was not paid for his work there.

At Christian Medical School, Murray operated on many disfigured patients. Some of his patients suffered from cleft lip or cleft palate. These birth defects cause a large gap, or cleft, in the patient's lip or the roof of the mouth. The defects make a person's face look strange. They can also make it hard for the person to speak or eat normally.

Murray also operated on patients who had been disfigured by leprosy. Leprosy is a disease that causes paralysis and loss of feeling in parts of the body, especially the face, hands, and feet. Many times, the damaged tissue rots away or must be removed. Murray reconstructed the faces and hands of leprosy patients to make their appearance more normal and help them live better lives.

After his return to Boston, Murray continued to perform plastic surgery and kidney transplants. He also performed research, wrote articles for medical journals, and traveled around the country giving speeches and presentations. However, he felt overwhelmed. He realized he had to decide where his true calling was.

Murray's work schedule was also hard on his family. Murray and Bobby had six children together: Meg, Ginny,

Tom, J. Link, Kathy, and Rick. However, Joseph Murray often spent long hours away from home, leaving Bobby to handle the day-to-day workings of the family and the household. Although Bobby and the children missed Murray, they knew that his dedication to his career and his patients was very important to him. Also, during the 1950s and 1960s, fathers were not as involved or "hands on" when it came to raising their children as they are today, so the family's situation was not unusual.

Although Murray was dedicated to his medical career, he made as much time for his family as he could. "Because of my hectic schedule, time with Bobby and the children was at a premium," he wrote in *Surgery of the Soul*. "One rule was held inviolate: we would take a family vacation for a full month every year." Every summer, the family went camping and hiking. They especially loved Chappaquiddick, an island off the coast of Massachusetts. In time, the Murrays bought land and built a simple house there, where they lived during their vacations.

It wasn't hard for Murray to choose plastic surgery as the type of medicine he wanted to concentrate on. "In my heart of hearts, I knew that the one aspect of my surgical life I could never give up was reconstructive plastic surgery," he wrote in *Surgery of the Soul*. In 1971 he resigned as Chief of Transplant Surgery at Brigham Hospital.

Many people were surprised at Murray's decision to give up transplant surgery in favor of plastic surgery. They believed that the two types of medicine were very different from each other. However, Murray felt that plastic surgery and transplants were more alike than different. Both involved using surgery to save or improve a person's life.

After all, performing plastic surgery on burn victims had introduced Murray to rejection and transplant surgery in the first place.

For the next 15 years, Murray performed many plastic surgery procedures. As with his earlier work, he especially enjoyed helping patients whose faces had been disfigured by cancer or birth defects.

Several of Murray's patients suffered from a birth defect called Crouzon's syndrome, which causes malformation of the face. A Crouzon's patient's eyes bulge out and his or her cheeks are sunken. The jaw is misshapen, so the teeth do not line up properly. To help Crouzon's patients, Murray studied a procedure first performed by a French doctor named Paul Tessier. He traveled to Paris, France, to observe Tessier operate on Crouzon's patients.

Tessier's procedure involved taking bone from other parts of the patient's body and grafting it to the bones of the face. Doing this allowed doctors to fill out the middle of the face so that the eyes, cheeks, and jaw were in their proper places. This delicate operation could take more than 12 hours and involve more than 80 separate steps. After Murray returned to Boston, he used Tessier's technique to help many Crouzon's patients.

In 1974 Murray once again brought his surgical skills to a faraway part of the world. In November he traveled to Tehran, Iran, to work for a month at Queen's Hospital. This hospital only treated patients who had been burned or who needed reconstructive surgery.

During his month in Tehran, Murray operated on many people. His patients were usually poor. They suffered from many different conditions. Some had tumors on their faces or had been injured in accidents. One of Murray's first patients there was a shepherd whose nose had been torn off by a wolf that attacked his flock of sheep.

Most of Murray's patients were children who had been terribly burned when they fell into the open pits used as ovens in many Iranian homes at that time. Murray didn't just perform operations to help these victims. He also taught the Iranian doctors on staff at the hospital. This meant that the doctors could continue to help patients after Murray returned home to the United States.

In his autobiography, Murray wrote about how important these foreign trips were to him. "Any doubts I might have had as to why I sometimes accepted these assignments abroad vanished during my first hospital rounds. Being exposed to patients with such stark, pressing needs was an eye-opening experience. . . . I felt that my lifetime of training had prepared me to come to this place. Aware that good fortune had bestowed on me a certain talent and superb education, I felt obliged to contribute my best to these patients. In so doing, I received far more than I gave. This was doctoring at its best!"

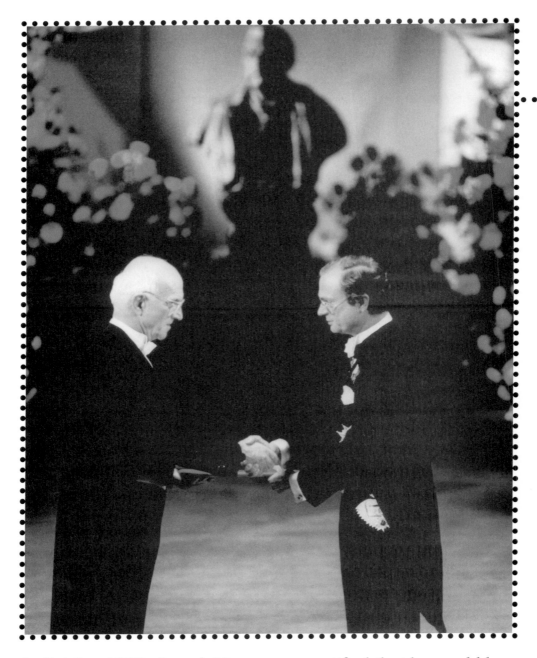

In October 1990, Joseph Murray was notified that he would be awarded the Nobel prize for medicine. Here he is shown receiving his award in Sweden.

Chapter 7
An Unexpected Event

• •

In 1986 Dr. Joseph Murray was 67 years old. He had been practicing medicine for 42 years. He'd had a long and successful career. Now he was ready for another part of his life. He decided to retire.

On March 20, just three months before he was scheduled to retire from his position at Brigham Hospital, Murray got up early and took a shower. As he washed, he thought about his busy schedule for the day. He had stayed up late the night before to write an article for a medical journal. That article still had to be finished. He also had to check his patients at the hospital. Then, later that day, he was going to fly down to the University of Alabama Medical School to give a series of lectures.

While he was in the shower, Murray's plans changed abruptly. His left leg felt weak. Then his left arm went numb. By the time he stumbled out of the shower, the left side of his face was tingling and he couldn't feel the fingers on his left hand.

Murray told Bobby that something was wrong. She called the doctor, then rushed Murray to Brigham Hospital. By four o'clock that afternoon, Murray was completely paralyzed on his left side. He had suffered a stroke.

A stroke happens when a blood vessel inside the brain either bursts or becomes blocked. The damaged vessel can no longer send oxygen-rich blood to part of the brain.

Without oxygen, the affected part of the brain may die. Usually, strokes affect one side of the body. The patient may be unable to move, feel anything, or talk. In severe strokes, the patient will go into a coma and may even die.

Although Murray's stroke was serious, he soon began to recover. By the next afternoon he was able to move his fingers. A few days later he was able to walk. Just one week after the stroke, Murray no longer felt numb anywhere on his body. However, he had to undergo several months of physical therapy in order to regain the full use of his left arm and leg. His doctors also insisted that he relax for six months. That meant he could not travel, give lectures, or practice medicine. So Murray retired a few months earlier than he had planned.

Murray recovered completely from his stroke. He also followed his doctors' advice about relaxing. Instead of practicing medicine and giving speeches, he read books, worked in the garden, and enjoyed spending time with his wife, six grown children, and many grandchildren.

In August 1990, Murray wrote a letter to his youngest son, Rick. He told Rick that he felt that the world had passed him by. Surely his contributions to surgery had already been forgotten.

Two months later, Murray would discover just how wrong he was.

In October 1990, Bobby and Joseph Murray were in California, visiting their daughter Meg. There they received some wonderful news. The Nobel Committee in Sweden had awarded the prize for medicine to Joseph Murray. Another doctor, E. Donnall Thomas, would share the prize with him. Thomas had also worked on transplants. He had researched the process of transplanting bone marrow cells.

Murray was surprised to receive the honor. He knew that he had been nominated for the Nobel Prize several times before. However, in 1988, three biochemists named George H. Hitchings, Gertrude B. Elion, and Sir James W. Black had been awarded the prize for their work in using drugs such as Imuran. The three scientists were honored for "their discoveries of important principles for drug treatment." Murray felt that this award acknowledged the use of drugs in successful kidney transplants, so he would never receive the award. Also, most of the Nobel Prize–winners were scientists who spent their time doing research. Very few were practicing physicians, as Murray was.

Two months later, Murray and his family traveled to Stockholm, Sweden. In an elegant and solemn ceremony on December 8, Murray received his award from the king and queen of Sweden. Murray called the ceremony "breathtaking." He also received a large cash prize. Murray donated the prize to Harvard Medical School, Brigham Hospital, and the Children's Hospital in Boston (where he had also performed many reconstructive surgeries) so that these institutions could continue their medical work.

Murray wrote an autobiography for the Nobel Prize committee. In it, he said: "We [his wife and he] have been blessed in our lives beyond my wildest dreams. My only wish would be to have ten more lives to live on this planet. If this were possible, I'd spend one lifetime each in embryology, genetics, physics, astronomy and geology. The other lifetimes would be as a pianist, backwoodsman, tennis player, or writer for the *National Geographic.* If anyone has bothered to read this far, you would note that I still have one future lifetime unaccounted for. That is because I'd like to keep open the option for another lifetime as a surgeon-scientist."

Although Murray actually spent more time performing plastic and reconstructive surgery than he did performing kidney transplants, his work in transplants changed medical science forever. During the 1950s, transplanting a kidney was a rare—and usually unsuccessful—event. Today, transplants have become fairly common. More than 20,000 transplants are performed every year. Most of these operations are kidney transplants. In addition, there are more than 20 different organs and tissues that can now be transplanted, including hearts, livers, lungs, corneas, and bone marrow. Countless lives have been improved or saved with these surgeries.

Joseph Murray's love for surgery shows in his dedication to his patients. Whether he was working to solve the mystery of kidney transplants or using his surgical skills to allow patients to look and feel better, he always used his medical training to give his patients a chance to live normal lives.

Joseph E. Murray Chronology

1919	Born in Milford, Massachusetts, on April 1
1936	Graduates from Milford High School
1940	Graduates from College of the Holy Cross
1943	Graduates from Harvard Medical School in December
1944-1947	Serves as staff surgeon at Valley Forge General Hospital
1945	Marries Virginia "Bobby" Link on June 2
1951	Begins practice as a plastic and general surgeon at Peter Bent Brigham Hospital in Boston (now Brigham and Women's Hospital)
1954	Performs the first successful human kidney transplant, using a kidney from a twin, on December 23
1962	Performs the first successful human kidney transplant using a kidney from a cadaver on April 5; spends two months working at the Christian Medical School in Vellore, India
1963	Publishes his first report on kidney transplants in the *New England Journal of Medicine*
1971	Resigns as Chief of Transplant Surgery at Brigham Hospital in order to focus on plastic and reconstructive surgery
1974	Works for a month at Queen's Hospital in Tehran, Iran
1986	Retires from his medical practice after suffering a stroke in March
1990	Receives the Nobel Prize in medicine

Transplant Timeline

1823	The first recorded report of transplant surgery occurs when German surgeon Carl Bunger grafts skin from a woman's thigh to her nose
1863	French scientist Paul Bert demonstrates that the body will reject foreign tissue
1903	German scientist Carl Jensen discovers that the body's immune system is responsible for tissue rejection
1905	Alexis Carrel develops techniques for rejoining severed blood vessels
1936	Dr. Voronoy, a Russian, reports the first human-to-human kidney transplant, when a kidney from a cadaver is transplanted to a recipient with a different blood type
1940s	Skin grafts are commonly used to treat burn victims and other seriously injured patients
1944	A British scientist, Sir Peter Medawar, reports that rejection of a transplant is based on immunologic factors. This discovery transforms transplant surgery from a largely unsuccessful operation to an accepted form of treatment

1954	Joseph Murray and John Hartwell Harrison perform the first successful human kidney transplant between identical twins
1959	Gertrude B. Elion develops the first drug that disrupts the body's immune system, 6-mercaptopurine
1962	Joseph Murray performs the first successful human kidney transplant using a kidney from a cadaver
1967	Thomas Starzl performs the first successful human liver transplant
1967	Christiaan Barnard performs the first successful human heart transplant
1968	Dr. Norman Shumway performs the first U.S. heart transplant at Stanford University
1972	Swiss scientist Jean Borel finds that the drug cyclosporine will suppress the immune system; it can prevent most cases of organ rejection
1983	Cyclosporine is approved for use in the United States
1994	The FDA approves Prograf (formerly FK506) for use in transplant recipients; marks a significant advance in the understanding and suppression of the human rejection response
1995	At Johns Hopkins Bayview Medical Center, Dr. Lloyd Ratner and Dr. Louis Kavoussi perform the world's first laparoscopic live-donor nephrectomy in which a patient's kidney is removed through a hole slightly larger than a silver dollar
1997	London Health Sciences Centre (London, Canada) transplants the liver, bowel, stomach, and pancreas into a 5-month-old infant, the world's youngest recipient of a multi-organ transplant

Further Reading

Books

Bankston, John. *Christaan Barnard and the Story of the First Successful Heart Transplant.* Bear, Del.: Mitchell Lane Publishers, 2002.

Curtis, Robert H., M.D. *Great Lives: Medicine.* New York: Charles Scribner's Sons, 1993.

Murray, Joseph E. *Surgery of the Soul.* Canton, Mass.: Science History Publications/USA, 2001.

Tracy, Kathleen. *Willem Kolff and the Invention of the Dialysis Machine.* Bear, Del.: Mitchell Lane Publishers, 2002.

On the Web

BBC Health
http://www.bbc.co.uk/health/immune/
History of Transplantation
http://www.livingbank.org/transplantation.html
Joseph E. Murray—Nobel Lecture
http://www.nobel.se/medicine/laureates/1990/murray-lecture.html
Kidshealth for Parents
http://www.kidshealth.org/parent/general/body_basics/
kidneys_urinary.html
A Science Odyssey: People and Discoveries: First Successful Kidney
Transplant Performed
http://www.pbs.org/wgbh/aso/databank/entries/dm54ki.html
Ten Nobels for the Future
http://www.hypothesis.it/nobel/eng/bio/murray.htm
TransWeb: All About Transplantation and Donation
http://www.transweb.org
Western Skies Dialysis Education Page
http://www.westernskiesdialysis.com/education/index.html

Glossary of Terms

acute   sudden and intense

allograft   a transplant taken from a body other than the recipient

appendectomy   the removal of a person's appendix

autograft   a transplant taken from the recipient's own body

cadaver   a dead body

chronic   a condition that lasts for a long time

creatinine waste material produced by muscles

donor   one who gives something, such as an organ, to another person

ethical   morally right

genetics   the study of ways that personal characteristics are passed from one generation to another

graft   tissue taken from one part of the body and used to repair damaged tissue on another part of the body

radiation tiny, harmful particles given off by certain materials

reconstruct   to rebuild something that has been damaged or destroyed

surgeon   a doctor who performs operations

toxic   poisonous

urea   waste material produced by the breakdown of proteins in the body

Index